ESSENTIAL OILS AND AROMATHERAPY

A complete guide on the use of natural essential oils and aromatherapy for promoting health, alleviating stress, enhancing beauty, inducing relaxation, and improving the home environment.

Dr. Amalie Kleist

Table of Contents

DISCLAIMER

This content is not meant to offer medical advice or replace advice or treatment from a personal physician. It is recommended that you get advice from your doctors or trained health specialists for any specific health inquiries you may have. Readers or followers of this instructional resource are responsible for any potential health effects.

Introduction

Dr. Amalie Kleist, a well-known holistic medicine specialist, introduces us to the realm of natural healing and wellbeing in "Essential Oils and Aromatherapy." In this interesting book, Dr. Kleist takes you on a trip through aromatherapy, an old healing method that uses essential oils to improve health, beauty, and mental health.

Dr. Kleist's extensive experience in clinical treatment and research contributes significantly to this thorough guide. Everything you need to know to utilize the therapeutic benefits of essential oils is covered in this book, from the history of aromatherapy to its useful applications and advanced methods. Learn about the healing properties of the purest essences found in nature as Dr. Kleist discusses the science of aromatherapy.

Learn how essential oils interact with the body and mind

to induce relaxation, decrease stress, and support general health. You'll find a plethora of natural solutions for daily wellbeing, ranging from treating common illnesses to improving mood and focus.

This book has something for everyone, regardless of your level of experience with essential oils or aromatherapy. Dr. Kleist offers concise, useful advice on choosing and utilizing essential oils in a secure and efficient manner. With simple recipes and recommendations for blending, diffusing, and topical application, you'll be able to make personalized aromatherapy mixes based on your own requirements and preferences.

However, "Essential Oils and Aromatherapy" is more than a practical handbook; it is a voyage of self-discovery and empowerment. Dr. Kleist encourages you to develop a feeling of harmony and balance in your life as well as a stronger connection to nature via mindfulness exercises, thought-provoking questions, and inspirational anecdotes. This book is your reliable guide to holistic well-being, whether your goals are to improve your beauty regimen, find relief from chronic pain, or just want a little peace of mind in an otherwise hectic environment. As you discover the incredible power of essential oils and set out on a life-changing path toward radiant health and energy, let Dr. Amalie Kleist be your guide.

"Essential Oils and Aromatherapy" is a guide to living a healthy, energetic, and prosperous life. It is more than simply a book. Today, embark on your adventure and discover the restorative properties of nature's scented treasures.

Chapter One

Introduction to Essential Oils and Aromatherapy

What are essential oils?

Plant extracts that are extremely concentrated are called essential oils. They encapsulate the "essence" of the health-promoting qualities and fragrance of the plant. Usually, these oils are extracted using techniques like distillation or cold pressing, which keep the plant's natural constituents intact. Aromatic molecules are what give essential oils their unique fragrances and medicinal qualities. For millennia, they have been utilized for their medicinal, cosmetic, and aromatic properties in a variety of cultures. Every essential oil has a distinct scent, chemical makeup, and possible health advantages of its own. They can be utilized in cleaning products, skincare, hair care, and aromatherapy, among other things.

What is Aromatherapy?

Aromatherapy is a comprehensive form of medicine that enhances mental, emotional, and physical health by utilizing the fragrant molecules found in plants, or essential oils. These concentrated plant extracts are used in a variety of ways, including diffusion, topical application, and inhalation.

The basis of aromatherapy is the theory that the fragrant substances in essential oils can interact with the limbic system, which is linked to emotions and memory, and the olfactory system, which is the body's sense of smell, to produce therapeutic benefits. These essential oils have the ability to cause physiological reactions when applied topically or inhaled, which can boost general health, reduce stress, elevate mood, and promote relaxation.

Aromatherapy is applied in a variety of situations, such as holistic medical settings, massage therapy sessions, spas, and even private homes. To maximize its benefits and advance a feeling of wellbeing, it is frequently combined with other complementary therapies, including massage therapy, yoga, and meditation. While using aromatherapy correctly is usually seen as safe, it's important to purchase high-quality essential oils, dilute them as needed, and be mindful of any potential allergies or sensitivities.

Aromatherapy methods can be customized to an individual's needs and preferences by consulting with a competent aromatherapist or healthcare practitioner.

How does Aromatherapy work?

Aromatherapy involves the inhalation or topical

application of aromatic compounds found in essential oils, which then interact with the body to produce therapeutic effects. Here's how it works:

- **INHALATION:** The volatile molecules in essential oils excite the olfactory nerves by passing via the nasal passages. The limbic system of the brain, which is involved in emotions, memory, and other processes, receives impulses from these nerves. Processing emotions and controlling bodily reactions are major functions of the limbic system. Essential oil inhalation can cause a range of physiological and mental reactions, including improved mood, stress relief, and relaxation.

- **CHEMICAL COMPOSITION:** Terpenes, phenols, and esters are only a few of the volatile molecules found in complex combinations found in essential oils. The scent and medicinal qualities of each essential oil are determined by its own distinct chemical composition. For instance, peppermint oil includes menthol, which has analgesic and cooling qualities, while lavender oil contains linalool and linalyl acetate, which are known for their calming and relaxing effects.

- **INDIVIDUAL VARIATION:** It's crucial to remember that each person will respond to aromatherapy differently based on their own sensitivity, health, and preferences, among other things. Certain essential oils or blends may have a stronger influence on certain people while having little or no impact on others.

- **TOPICAL APPLICATION:** You can use essential oils topically to absorb them into your skin and bloodstream. After being absorbed, the chemicals in the essential oils interact with cells and organs all over the body, as well as receptors in the skin and underlying tissues. This may result in both systemic benefits like relaxation or immunological support and localized benefits like pain alleviation or skin rejuvenation.

- **SYNERGISTIC BENEFITS:** Several chemicals found in essential oils frequently combine to create therapeutic benefits in a synergistic way. This indicates that these substances have a bigger overall effect than the sum of their separate actions. For instance, combining essential oils like chamomile and lavender may have a more powerfully soothing impact than using just one oil.

Overall, by inhalation or topical application, aromatherapy uses the potent aromatic molecules in essential oils to support overall well-being, enhance mood, relieve stress, and encourage relaxation.

Chapter Two

Understanding Essential Oils

Methods for extracting essential oils: Advantages and Disadvantages

Different techniques are used to extract essential oils from plants, depending on the kind of plant material and the final product that is intended. Here are a few typical extraction techniques:

Steam distillation

This is one of the most frequent ways to extract essential oils from aromatic plants. Steam is used in steam distillation to evaporate the essential oils from the plant material. After that, the steam and vaporized essential oil are separated and condensed back into liquid form. A large variety of plant components, such as flowers, leaves, and stems, can be processed with this technique.

> **Advantages:**

- Gentle process that protects the plant's sensitive, fragrant ingredients.

- It is suitable for a variety of plant materials, such as stems, leaves, and flowers.

- Minimum deterioration while producing essential oils of superior quality.

> **Disadvantages:**

- It uses copious amounts of water and plant material.

- During distillation, some chemicals that are sensitive to heat could be lost.

- The process can take a long time and calls for specific tools.

Hydrodistillation

Boiling the plant material in water is the method used in this version of steam distillation. The essential oils are extracted from the plant material by the steam that is created, and they are then gathered and separated from the water in a condenser. Essential oils are frequently extracted from woody or resinous plant components using this technique.

➤ **Advantages:**

- This product is perfect for removing oil from woody or resinous plant materials.

- This is an easy and conventional technique that requires little in the way of equipment.

- Able to generate superior-quality essential oils.

➤ **Disadvantages:**

- It requires a lot of plant material and water.

- In comparison to steam distillation, the process might be cumbersome and ineffective.

- During distillation, heat-sensitive chemicals could break down.

Solvent Extraction

This method is used to extract essential oils from plant materials, like fragile flowers that are unsuitable for steam distillation. This process involves dissolving the essential oils from the plant material in a solvent, usually hexane or ethanol. The concentrated essential oil extract is then removed by evaporating the solvent. Even if solvent extraction is efficient, the finished product may contain traces of solvent residues.

➤ **Advantages:**

- This is an effective technique for removing oil from fragile plants and flowers.

- The plant is able to provide significant essential oil outputs.

- Ideal for extracting fragrance-dense oils.

➢ **Disadvantages:**

- The process may leave behind residual solvents in the finished product, which, if improperly eliminated, may be hazardous.

- It requires handling volatile chemicals with caution.

- There is a possibility of heat-induced aromatic compound breakdown during solvent evaporation.

Carbon Dioxide (CO2) Extraction

This relatively new technique extracts essential oils from

plant material by applying high pressure to carbon dioxide. This process compresses carbon dioxide to the point that it forms a supercritical fluid, which combines the characteristics of a gas and a liquid. The essential oils are then extracted using this supercritical CO2, producing an excellent extract with no thermal damage to the aromatic components.

➤ **Advantages:**

- It produces extracts of superior quality with no heat damage.

- This is an adaptable technique that works with a variety of plant materials.

- It is environmentally beneficial because CO2 is widely available and non-toxic.

➤ **Disadvantages:**

- The task requires specific tools and knowledge, which increases the expense.

- Delicate aromatic compounds can be impacted by high temperatures and pressures.

- The process can demand a lot of energy and time.

Expression or Cold Pressing

This method is most commonly employed to extract essential oils from citrus fruits, including lemon, orange, and grapefruit. To extract the essential oils, the fruit rinds are mechanically pressed. Because cold pressing doesn't use heat, unlike steam distillation, the delicate aromatic components in the oils are preserved.

➢ **Advantages:**

- It does not use heat, conserving the volatile components in the oils.

- Easy and uncomplicated procedure.

- It is ideal for taking the oil out of citrus fruits.

> **Disadvantages:**

- It only works with plant parts that have a lot of oil, like orange rinds.

- Lower yields may be obtained as compared to other approaches.

- It necessitates mechanical pressure, which can be laborious.

Enfleurage

Enfleurage is a traditional technique mostly used to extract essential oils from fragile flowers like tuberose and jasmine. Using this technique, the flowers are placed on a layer of fat, such as vegetable or animal oil, which gradually absorbs the fragrant components. The essential oils are then removed from the fat by washing it with alcohol, leaving behind a highly aromatic oil called "pomade."

> **Advantages:**

- Ideal for removing oil from fragile flowers that have been harmed by heat.

- The conventional method preserves the inherent scent of the flowers.

- Able to yield oils with a strong scent.

> **Disadvantages:**

- This is a labor-intensive procedure that requires the oil or fat to be changed frequently.

- The process is limited to small-scale manufacturing due to its time-consuming nature.

- Because it requires a lot of labor, the finished oils could be costly.

The choice of extraction method is based on various aspects, including the type of plant material, the desired end result, and the quality of the final extract. Each extraction method has its own advantages and disadvantages.

Carrier oils: Their function and significance

Carrier oils are important in aromatherapy because they dilute essential oils and act as a medium for safe skin application. Carrier oils play important parts, which are listed below:

Safety: By serving as a barrier to shield the skin from irritation, burning, or allergic responses, carrier oils help to keep essential oils safe. They do no damage and help "carry" the essential oils onto the skin's surface to aid in their absorption.

Dilution: Undiluted application of essential oils, which are extremely concentrated extracts, may cause skin irritation or sensitization. Carrier oils aid in the dilution of essential oils, lowering the possibility of negative responses while maintaining the essential oils' ability to penetrate the skin and work their magic.

Absorption: The aromatic ingredients and medicinal qualities of essential oils are released more gradually thanks to carrier oils' slower rate of skin absorption than those of essential oils. This extended absorption lengthens the effects of aromatherapy and encourages a more profound state of relaxation.

Versatility: Carrier oils are adaptable supplements to any skincare or health regimen since they can be used as massage oils or moisturizers on their own. Additionally, they can serve as the foundation for DIY skincare products like creams, lotions, and balms.

Customization: Essential oils and carrier oils can be combined to make skincare products, massage oils, and aromatherapy blends that are specific to each person's requirements and tastes. Numerous combinations and compositions are possible since different carrier oils each have special qualities and advantages.

Moisturization: The fatty acids, vitamins, and other nutrients found in carrier oils help to moisturize and nourish the skin. They prevent dryness and encourage smooth, soft skin by supporting the preservation of the skin's moisture barrier.

Slip and glide: carrier oils are perfect for topical and massage treatments because of their lubricating qualities. Their flowing, silky texture makes them easy to apply and lessens discomfort and friction during massage.

Stability: Over time, carrier oils help keep essential oils stable by preventing oxidation and degradation. They serve as organic preservatives, maintaining the strength and efficacy of essential oil blends while increasing their shelf life.

All things considered, carrier oils are fundamental to aromatherapy because they offer a flexible, safe, and efficient method of applying essential oils to medical conditions. Carrier oils are an integral part of any aromatherapy practice, whether they are utilized for dilution, moisturization, massage, or customization.

Chapter Three

Common essential oils with their potential benefits

Lavender oil

It is very beneficial and gentle. It has multiple applications. Try adding it to a bath or diffuser as aromatherapy, adding it to water to produce a room spray or body spritzer, or combining it with a base oil to make body oil. Lavender helps alleviate stress, pain and promote sleep.

According to studies, before the discovery of antiseptics, lavender was used as a hospital cleaning agent.

Studies have also indicated that the use of tea tree and lavender oils may disrupt young boys' hormones.

Tea tree oil

Tea tree oil is commonly used as an antifungal, antiseptic, and antibacterial. It can also be helpful in the following ways:

Acne: Dip a cotton swab into tea tree essential oil. Apply it directly to the acne; this is one instance in which dilution is unnecessary. It can help you get rid of acne faster.

Athlete's foot and ringworms: Mix it with a carrier oil, which is a base or vegetable oil like coconut or jojoba oil that helps dilute essential oils, and then apply it to the skin to treat it.

Eucalyptus oil

Keeping eucalyptus essential oil on hand is a good idea during the colder months. It improves your breathing by widening your nasal airways and relieving nasal stuffiness. (Peppermint oil could also be effective in this situation.) Its antibacterial and anti-inflammatory properties aid in combating the herpes simplex virus and alleviating discomfort. Use eucalyptus oil with caution and dilute it before applying it topically. It can have negative effects on children and pets and should not be consumed.

Frankincense oil

Frankincense, known as the "king of oils," improves mood, sleep, and inflammation. According to some research, it may also help prevent gum disease and asthma. Frankincense oil's woody, spicy perfume makes it a popular element in skin treatments and can also be used in aromatherapy. Before applying frankincense oil to your skin, ensure it is diluted.

Peppermint oil

Peppermint oil has been known to:

- Contains antibacterial, antifungal, and anti-inflammatory properties.

- Relieve headaches.

- Combat fatigue.

- Lift your spirits.

- Reduce intestinal spasms.

- Aid digestion.

- Enhance memory.

Always dilute the oil before using it topically.

Cedarwood oil

Cedarwood oil, known for its pleasant woody scent, is a popular component in deodorants, shampoos, and insect repellents due to its antioxidant and antibacterial properties. However, cedarwood oil can also be used to alleviate anxiety and sleeplessness. Cedarwood oil, when blended with a carrier oil, can be used directly or in aromatherapy.

Lemon oil

Lemon oil is derived from lemon peels and may be applied topically to the skin with a carrier oil or diffused into the air. The use of lemon oil demonstrated:

- Reduces stress and depression.

- Reduce pain.

- Reduce nausea.

- Destroy germs.

According to one research, aromatherapy with essential oils, such as lemon oil, may improve Alzheimer's patients' cognitive abilities. Lemon oil is safe to use both topically and aromatically.

On the other hand, there are studies that claim that lemon oil might make your skin more vulnerable to the sun, which could lead to a higher risk of sunburn. After applying, keep yourself out of direct sunlight. Some of these include lemon, lime, orange, grapefruit, lemongrass, and bergamot oils.

Bergamot oil

The fruity and flowery-smelling oil can be used topically with a carrier oil or diffused (though it may induce photosensitivity).

Bergamot oil is known for its ability to:

- Reduce anxiety.

- Improve mood.

- Lower blood pressure.

Lemongrass oil

Lemongrass oil, with its strong citrus scent, is well-known for its ability to relieve stress, anxiety, and despair. Its antimicrobial properties make it an effective natural remedy for healing wounds and eradicating infections. It has been shown to inhibit the growth of the fungi that cause jock itch, ringworm, and athlete's foot. According to research, lemongrass oil can help people with type 2 diabetes reduce their blood sugar levels. Before applying it to your skin, be sure you use a carrier oil.

Orange oil

Orange oil is extracted from the rinds of citrus fruits. It

can be applied directly to the skin (with a carrier oil), diffused into the air, or used as a natural household cleaner.

Orange oil has been recognized for:

- Germs elimination

- Decreasing anxiety

- Reducing pain.

Applying orange oil to your skin and then going outdoors should be done with caution, because it might make your skin more sensitive to sunlight.

Rosemary oil

You've most certainly used rosemary to enhance the flavor of some of your dishes. However, there are also benefits to using rosemary oil, such as improved mental clarity, increased hair development, reduced stress and discomfort, elevated mood, and reduced joint inflammation. When mixed with a carrier oil, rosemary oil is safe to apply straight to the skin or use in aromatherapy. We don't advocate taking rosemary oil if you have high blood pressure, epilepsy, or are pregnant.

10 unique DIY essential oil recipes for a variety of uses

Citrus-Refreshing Room Spray:

- 10 drops of sweet orange essential oil.

- 5 drops of lemon essential oil.

- 5 drops of grapefruit essential oil.

- Distilled water.

In a 4-ounce spray bottle, add the essential oils and top it off with distilled water. Shake thoroughly before each use, then spray across the room for a fresh and revitalizing smell.

Pillow Mist for Deep Sleep:

- 10 drops of lavender essential oil.

- 5 drops of chamomile essential oil

- 3 drops of cedarwood essential oil

- 2 oz. distilled water

In a 2-ounce spray bottle, add the essential oils and top it off with distilled water. Shake thoroughly before each use, then lightly spritz your pillow and sheets before bedtime for a peaceful night's sleep.

Calming Scalp Therapy:

- 3 drops of tea tree essential oil

- 3 drops of lavender essential oil

- 2 drops of peppermint essential oil

- 2 tablespoons of coconut oil

To relieve irritation, encourage healthy hair, and lessen dandruff, combine the essential oils with coconut oil and massage the mixture into the scalp.

Bath Soak for Muscle Relief:

- 5 drops of eucalyptus essential oil

- 5 drops of peppermint essential oil

- 3 drops of rosemary essential oil

- 1 cup Epsom salt

Thoroughly combine the essential oils with the Epsom salt. To ease tense and painful muscles, add the mixture to a warm bath and soak for 20 to 30 minutes.

Inhaler Blend for Mood Enhancement:

- 5 drops of bergamot essential oil

- 5 drops of lemon essential oil

- 3 drops of geranium essential oil

- Cotton wick inhaler

Fill the inhaler's cotton wick with essential oils, then slide it into the inhaler tube. Every time you need a mood boost or an energy boost, take a deep inhalation.

Relaxing Massage Oil:

- 5 drops of lavender essential oil

- 5 drops of frankincense essential oil

- 3 drops of cedarwood essential oil

- 2 tablespoons of sweet almond oil

Blend sweet almond oil with essential oils to create a relaxing massage oil that helps soothe the body and mind.

Pure insect repellent spray:

- 10 drops of citronella essential oil

- 5 drops of eucalyptus essential oil

- 5 drops of lavender essential oil

- 2 ounces of witch hazel

Fill a 2-ounce spray bottle with witch hazel and add the essential oils. Before use, give it a thorough shake, then spray on the skin and clothes to ward off insects like mosquitoes and so on.

Homemade Beard Oil:

- 5 drops of cedarwood essential oil

- 5 drops of sandalwood essential oil

- 3 drops of peppermint essential oil

- 2 tablespoons of jojoba oil

Apply a mixture of essential oils and jojoba oil to the beard to soften, condition, and encourage healthy growth.

All-natural Floor Cleaner:

- 10 drops of lemon essential oil

- 5 drops of tea tree essential oil

- 3 drops of lavender essential oil

- 1 cup of white vinegar

- 2 cups of water

Put all the contents into a spray bottle and use it to naturally clean and disinfect floors.

Roller Blend for headache relief:

- 5 drops of peppermint essential oil

- 3 drops of lavender essential oil

- 2 drops of chamomile essential oil

- 10 mL roller bottle

Fill the roller bottle halfway with fractionated coconut oil and add the essential oils. For natural headache treatment, apply to the neck, forehead, and temples.

Before utilizing a new essential oil combination, always conduct a patch test, particularly if you have sensitive skin. Depending on the size of the container you're using and your own tastes, adjust the quantity of drops. Take advantage of these homemade essential oil recipes.

Chapter Four

Aromatherapy methods and applications.

Aromatherapy is a holistic medical practice that enhances mental, emotional, and physical health by using essential oils—natural plant extracts. The following are some methods and uses for aromatherapy:

INHALATION: One of the most popular ways to use essential oils in aromatherapy is by inhalation. You may accomplish this by taking a whiff of a few drops of essential oil, adding the oil to a bowl of hot water, and then inhaling the steam, or you can just inhale straight from the bottle.

COMPRESSES: Aromatherapy compresses are made by soaking a cloth in a blend of water and essential oils before applying it to the skin. Skin ` problems, inflammation, and localized discomfort are frequently treated using this technique.

MASSAGE: Aromatherapy massage combines the calming effects of a massage treatment with the therapeutic effects of essential oils. During a massage, diluted essential oils are applied to the skin, where they are absorbed and offer a number of psychological and physical advantages.

BATHS: A warm bath enhanced with a few drops of essential oils may be opulent and healing. While the steam enables inhalation, the water's heat aids in releasing the oils' fragrance. Taking a bath with essential oils can help with skin health, relaxation, and muscular release.

STEAM INHALATION: This method includes placing a towel over the head to form a tent while a few drops of essential oil are added to a bowl of hot water. After that, the user takes a deep breath of the steam, which helps relieve headaches, sinus problems, and lung congestion.

TOPICAL APPLICATION: By diluting essential oils with a carrier oil (such as coconut, almond, or jojoba oil), the oils can be administered topically via massage, compresses, or baths. By doing this, the therapeutic properties of the oils may be absorbed via the skin and into the bloodstream.

SPRAYS AND MISTS: Essential oils may be used to make face mists or room sprays by diluting them with water. These can be used as a portable aromatherapy sampler, to refresh the air, or to create a relaxing ambiance.

DIFFUSION: Aromatherapy diffusers are gadgets that release essential oils into the atmosphere to facilitate inhalation and produce a relaxing environment. There are many different kinds of diffusers out there, such as nebulizing, reed, and ultrasonic diffusers.

It's crucial to use pure, high-quality essential oils for aromatherapy and to dilute them appropriately before applying them to the skin. Before using essential oils, it's also important to take into account any contraindications or potential allergies, especially for children, pregnant women, and those with certain medical problems.

Ratios of dilution and Safety measures

RATIOS OF DILUTION

For topical use: Adults: A typical dilution ratio is 2-3%, which means 2-3 drops of essential oil for every teaspoon (5 mL) of carrier oil.

For little children, the elderly, or people with sensitive

skin, a dilution ratio of 1% or less is advised. Typically, this means 1 essential oil drop for every teaspoon of carrier oil.

For Inhalation: The manner of inhaling might affect the dilution ratios. It is common practice to add 3–7 drops of essential oil to a bowl of hot water for steam inhalation.

Regarding diffusion, abide by the directions provided by the manufacturer for the particular diffuser being utilized.

SAFETY MEASURES

Patch Test: Prior to utilizing any essential oil topically, always do a patch test. To test for any negative responses, apply a small quantity of diluted oil to a small area of skin (such as the inner forearm) and wait 24 hours.

Phototoxicity: When exposed to sunshine or UV radiation, some essential oils, particularly citrus oils like bergamot, lime, and lemon, can trigger phototoxic responses and skin irritation. After using these oils topically, stay out of the sun.

Skin Sensitivity: Because essential oils are strong, they may irritate or sensitize the skin, particularly when used topically or in large quantities. Prior to applying essential oils to the skin, always dilute them with a carrier oil.

Pregnancy and Health Issues: Before using essential oils, those with certain medical issues, the elderly, children, pregnant women, nursing mothers, and other caregivers should speak with a trained healthcare provider. There are circumstances or phases of pregnancy where specific essential oils should not be used.

Quality and Purity: To guarantee safety and efficacy, choose pure, premium essential oils from reliable suppliers. Steer clear of synthetic or contaminated oils since they could not have the same therapeutic effects and might have unfavorable side effects.

Storage and Handling: To maintain the effectiveness of essential oils, store them in dark glass bottles in a cool, dark area away from heat sources and direct sunlight. Keep children and pets away from essential oils.

Respiratory Sensitivity: Exercise caution while inhaling some essential oils, particularly if you have allergies or asthma. Powerful oils such as peppermint or eucalyptus can be overpowering and may worsen respiratory complaints if breathed in excess.

It will be easier to guarantee safe and satisfying aromatherapy encounters if you abide by these dilution ratios and safety measures. It's always preferable to speak with a licensed aromatherapist or other healthcare provider if you have particular health concerns or inquiries about utilizing essential oils.

Chapter Five

Aromatherapy for well-being and health

Aromatherapy is a holistic therapeutic technique that uses natural plant extracts, known as essential oils, to enhance health and well-being. These essential oils, which are derived from a variety of plant components, including fruits, leaves, stems, roots, and flowers, contain the aromatic molecules that give plants their distinct fragrances. The following are some ways that aromatherapy promotes wellbeing and health:

SKIN CARE: The antibacterial and anti-inflammatory qualities of essential oils, such as those found in tea tree, lavender, and chamomile, can help the skin. Applying these oils topically can help cure acne, relieve irritated skin, and improve the general health of the skin when diluted with a carrier oil.

STRESS REDUCTION: A number of essential oils, including bergamot, lavender, and chamomile, are well-known for their ability to induce calmness and relaxation. These oils can be used in massages or inhaled to help lower tension and anxiety levels.

MOOD ENHANCEMENT: Essential oils have the potential to improve mood. Orange and lemon essential oils are examples of uplifting citrus oils that may boost vitality and uplift one's spirit. The stimulating properties of peppermint oil might help improve attention and alertness.

IMMUNE SUPPORT: The antibacterial qualities of some essential oils, such as those of tea tree, eucalyptus, and oregano, can help support and guard against infections. These oils can help cleanse the air and stop the spread of airborne diseases when diffused in the air or used as a room spray.

ENHANCED SLEEP: One of lavender oil's most well-known uses is to encourage calm and enhance the quality of one's sleep. Improved sleep can be facilitated by diffusing lavender oil in the bedroom or by adding a few drops to a warm bath prior to bed.

RESPIRATORY HEALTH: Breathing in essential oils has a positive impact on respiratory health as well. Essential oils with decongestant qualities, such as peppermint and eucalyptus, can help open up nasal passages and ease the symptoms of respiratory ailments, including sinusitis and colds.

PAIN RELIEF: Due to their analgesic qualities, certain essential oils, such as peppermint and eucalyptus, can help reduce aches and pains in the muscles. These oils can be massaged into the afflicted region or administered topically after being diluted in a carrier oil.

It's crucial to remember that aromatherapy cannot replace medical care; rather, it can be a complimentary therapy for enhancing health and wellness. Before using essential oils, it is always a good idea to speak with a licensed healthcare provider, particularly if you are pregnant, nursing or have any underlying medical concerns.

Furthermore, because essential oils are extremely concentrated materials, they should be used carefully, diluted appropriately, and kept out of the eyes and mucous membranes.

Integrating aromatherapy into everyday life

Including aromatherapy in your daily routine may be an easy and fun method to support general wellbeing and health. The following are some suggestions for including aromatherapy into your everyday schedule:

- **Begin Your Day with a Positive Scent:** Use citrus essential oils, such as those from lemon, orange, or grapefruit, in a diffuser to set the mood for energy in the morning. You might feel more cheerful and refreshed for the rest of the day when you inhale the crisp, energizing scent.

- **Use Aromatherapy in Your Meditation or Yoga Practice:** Diffusing grounding essential oils, such as sandalwood, patchouli, or frankincense, during yoga or meditation sessions might improve your mindfulness practice. A deeper and more fulfilling practice may be made possible by the earthy and balancing scents, which can aid in fostering a sense of peace and concentration.

- **Make Natural Cleaning Solutions:** Make your

own non-toxic cleaning solutions with antimicrobial essential oils such as tea tree, lemon, or lavender. White vinegar and water may be combined with a few drops of your preferred essential oil to create a multipurpose cleanser that leaves surfaces clean and fragrant.

- **Employ Aromatherapy in Your Workspace:** To improve focus, attention, and productivity while working, place a little diffuser on your desk and fill it with essential oils such as eucalyptus, rosemary, or peppermint. These energizing aromas can support your continuous alertness and renewal throughout the day.

- **Use Aromatherapy While Working Out:** Place a moist towel next to your exercise area and add a few drops of energetic essential oils, such as peppermint or eucalyptus. During workouts, the energizing scent may help boost motivation and toughness.

- **Take Aromatherapy on the Go:** When traveling, carry your preferred essential oils in a compact diffuser or inhaler. Aromatherapy can help reduce stress associated with travel, encourage relaxation, and foster a sense of familiarity and comfort in strange places—whether you're in a hotel room, on a train, or in an airplane.

- **Personal Care Regimen:** Use a few drops of essential oils in your body wash, moisturizer, or shampoo to include them in your regimen. In addition to giving your everyday grooming regimen a natural and fragrant boost, essential oils like tea tree, lavender, and rosemary can also support healthy skin and hair.

- **Establish a Calm Bedtime Routine:** Unwind in your bedroom at night by diffusing essential oils that promote relaxation, such as lavender, chamomile, or cedarwood. To encourage relaxation and enhance the quality of your sleep, you can also add a few drops of lavender oil to a warm bath or combine it with another oil for a calming massage right before bed.

You may enjoy the many advantages of essential oils and improve your general health and well-being by implementing aromatherapy into your everyday life in these easy ways.

Chapter Six

Special concerns and safety measures: aromatherapy and pregnancy, aromatherapy for kids

Due to the inherent sensitivities and vulnerabilities of pregnant women and children, there are some additional concerns and safety measures to bear in mind when utilizing aromatherapy during pregnancy.

AROMATHERAPY AND PREGNANCY:

➤ *Speak with a Healthcare Professional:* Before taking any essential oils while pregnant, it's imperative that you speak with your healthcare practitioner. Certain essential oils may be contraindicated or call for extra care, however, many essential oils are usually regarded as safe when taken correctly during pregnancy.

➢ *Select Safe Essential Oils:* Lavender, chamomile, ylang-ylang, and citrus oils like lemon and orange are among the essential oils that are thought to be safe to use during pregnancy. However, because they may cause contractions, oils like clary sage, rosemary, and basil should be avoided when pregnant.

➢ *Dilution and Inhalation:* During pregnancy, essential oils should be utilized at low dilutions (usually 1% or less). Diffusing or putting a few drops on a cotton ball or tissue by inhalation is typically seen as a safer mode of administration than topical use, particularly in the first trimester when the risk of miscarriage is at its maximum.

➢ *Avoid Internal Use:* Unless directed by a licensed healthcare provider, pregnant women should refrain from consuming essential oils. Certain oils can be harmful if consumed, which puts the mother and the unborn child in danger.

➤ *Keep an Eye Out for Sensitivities:* Being pregnant might make you more sensitive to particular scents, so pay attention to how you respond to certain essential oils. If you feel uncomfortable or have any negative reactions, stop using the product and speak with your doctor.

AROMATHERAPY FOR KIDS:

➤ *Age Appropriateness:* Children can safely use aromatherapy, but it's important to take into account their age and developmental stage. Because certain oils are so strong, they might not be appropriate for infants or young children.

➤ *Select Child-Friendly Oils:* Use essential oils such as lavender, chamomile, mandarin, and tea tree that are mild and suitable for young people when utilizing aromatherapy. Extreme oils, such as eucalyptus or peppermint, should not be used on young children due to their extreme potency, which might irritate their respiratory systems.

➢ *Correct Dilution:* Before putting essential oils on a child's skin, they should always be diluted. For children, the suggested dilution ratio is usually between 0.25% and 1%, which is substantially lower than for adults. Dilution is frequently accomplished with carrier oils such as sweet almond or coconut oil.

➢ *Patch Test:* To rule out any potential allergic reactions or sensitivities, test a tiny area of the skin with diluted essential oils before applying them to a larger area.

➢ *Caution while Inhaling:* Because infants' and

young children's respiratory systems are still growing and may be more sensitive to strong scents, exercise caution when diffusing essential oils around them. Use the diffuser sparingly for brief periods of time and keep it in a well-ventilated location.

➤ *Safety Storage:* To avoid inadvertent consumption or misuse, keep aromatherapy items and essential oils out of children's reach. Keep them in a cool, dark area, out of direct sunlight and heat.

You may safely enjoy the positive benefits of aromatherapy during pregnancy and with children while reducing any potential hazards or negative responses by taking special concerns and safety measures.

ACKNOWLEDGEMENTS

All glory belongs to God. I'd also want to thank my wonderful family, partner, fans, readers, friends, and customers for their constant support and words of encouragement.

www.ingramcontent.com/pod-product-compliance
Lightning Source LLC
Chambersburg PA
CBHW031134020426
42333CB00012B/379